The Air Fryer Toaster Oven Lunch Recipe Collection

Boost Your Metabolism And Enjoy Your Meals With Incredibly Tasty Air Fryer Toaster Oven Dishes

Eva Morris

TABLE OF CONTENT

Hot Flank Steaks With Roasted Peanuts...7

Authentic Wiener Beef Schnitzel.. 9

Dreamy Beef Steak With Rice, Broccoli And Green Beans........ 10

Mustard Pork Chops With Lemon Zest.......................................12

Herbed Beef Roast.. 15

Roast Pork Belly With Cumin...17

Sunday Night Garlic Beef Schnitzel..19

Meatballs With Parsley And Thyme... 21

Garlic Lamb Chops With Thyme...23

Ginger Rack Rib Steak.. 25

Cheeseburger Egg Rolls..27

Air Fried Grilled Steak.. 29

Juicy Cheeseburgers.. 30

Spicy Thai Beef Stir-Fry..32

Beef Brisket Recipe From Texas..35

Copycat Taco Bell Crunch Wraps... 37

Air Fryer Beef Casserole... 39

Meat Lovers' Pizza.. 41

Chimichurri Skirt Steak... 44

Country Fried Steak..46

Italian Meatballs...48

Lamb Chops With Rosemary Sauce.....................................50

Roast Lamb Shoulder.. 53

Garlicky Lamb Chops...55

New England Lamb.. 57

Onion Lamb Kebabs.. 60

Zucchini Lamb Meatballs...63

Mint Lamb With Roasted Hazelnuts.............................. 66

Lamb Rack With Lemon Crust......................................68

Braised Lamb Shanks.. 71

Za'atar Lamb Chops.. 73

Simple Beef Sirloin Roast..76

Seasoned Beef Roast...79

Bacon-Wrapped Filet Mignon...................................... 81

Beef Burgers.. 83

Beef Jerky... 88

Sweet & Spicy Meatballs.. 91

Spiced Pork Shoulder..95

Seasoned Pork Tenderloin.. 99

Basil Meatloaf With Parmesan.....................................102

Homemade Beef Liver Soufflé..................................... 104

Rib Eye Steak With Avocado Sauce...............................105

medical or professional advice. The content within this book has been derived from various sources. Please consult a licensed professional before attempting any techniques outlined in this book.

By reading this document, the reader agrees that under no circumstances is the author responsible for any losses, direct or indirect, which are incurred as a result of the use of information contained within this document, including, but not limited to, — errors, omissions, or inaccuracies.

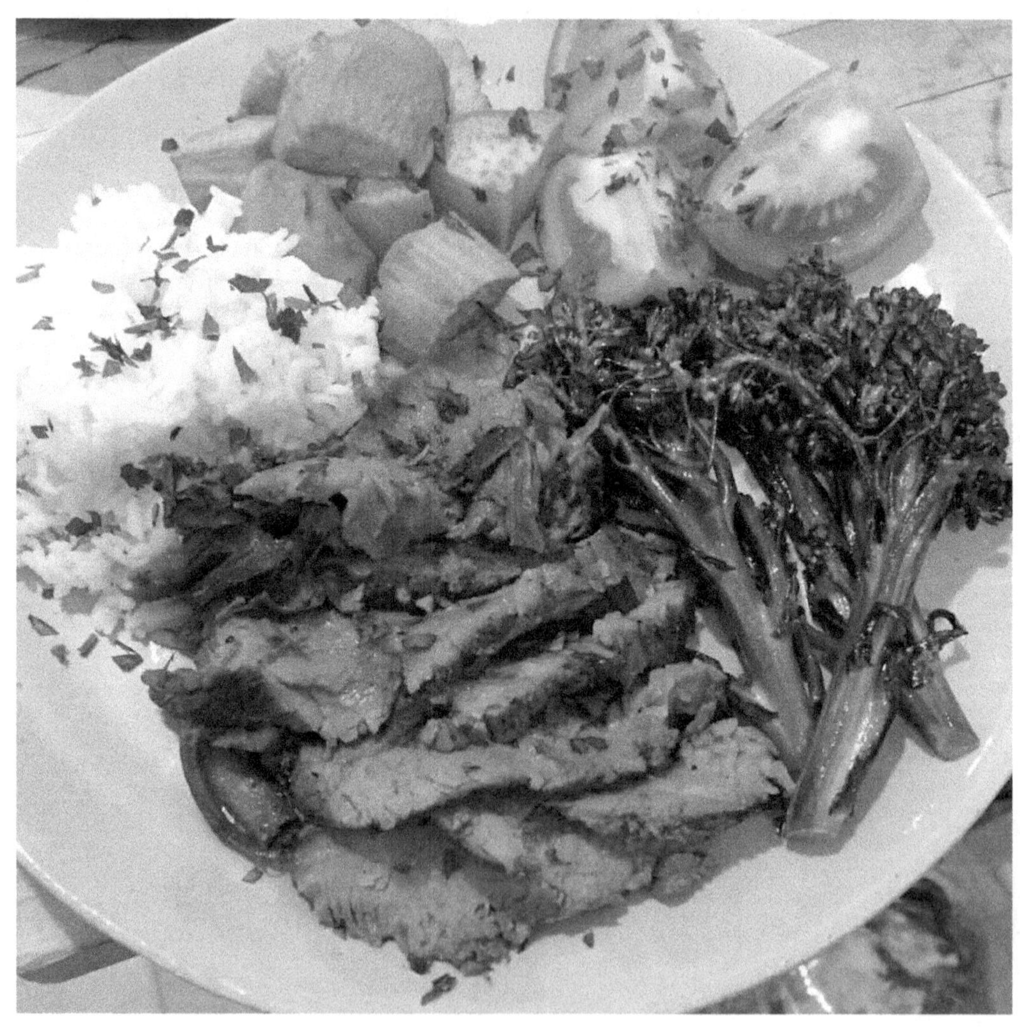

Hot Flank Steaks With Roasted Peanuts

Preparation Time: 10minutes

Cooking time: 35 minutes

Servings: 3 to 4

Ingredients:

- 2 lb. flank steaks, cut into long strips

- 2 tbsp. fish sauce

- 2 tbsp. soy sauce

- 2 tbsp. sugar

- 2 tbsp. ground garlic

- 2 tbsp. ground ginger

- 2 tsp. hot sauce

- 1 cup chopped cilantro, divided into two

- ½ cup roasted peanuts, chopped

Directions:

1. Preheat the Air Fryer to 400 F. In a zipper bag, add the beef, fish sauce, swerve sweetener, garlic, soy sauce, ginger, half of the cilantro, and hot sauce. Zip the bag

and massage the Ingredients: with your hands to mix well.

2. Open the bag, remove the beef, shake off the excess marinade, place the beef strips in the fryer basket in a single layer, and avoid overlapping. Close the Air Fryer and cook for 5 minutes.

3. Turn the beef and cook further for 5 minutes.

4. Dish the cooked meat in a serving platter, garnish with the peanuts and the remaining cilantro.

Authentic Wiener Beef Schnitzel

Preparation Time: 10 minutes

Cooking Time: 25 minutes

Serving: 4

Ingredients:

- 4beef schnitzel cutlets
- ½ cup flour
- 2eggs, beaten
- Salt and black pepper
- 1cup breadcrumbs

Directions:

1. Coat the cutlets in flour and shake off any excess. Dip the coated cutlets into the beaten egg. Sprinkle with salt and black pepper. Then dip into the crumbs and to cover well. Spray them generously with oil and cook for 10 minutes at 360 F, turning once halfway through.

Dreamy Beef Steak With Rice, Broccoli And Green Beans

Preparation Time: 40 minutes

Servings: 2

Ingredients:

- 1lb beef steak,
- Salt and black pepper to taste to season

Fried Rice:

- 2½ cups of rice
- 1½ tbsp. soy sauce
- 2tsp sesame oil
- 2tsp minced ginger
- 2tsp vinegar
- One clove garlic, minced
- ¼ cup chopped broccoli
- ¼ cup green beans

Directions:

1. Put the beef on a chopping board and use a knife to cut it into 2-inch strips. Add the meat to a bowl, sprinkle with pepper and salt, and mix it with a spoon. Let it sit for 10 minutes. Preheat the Air Fryer to 400 F. Add the beef to the fryer basket, and cook for 5 minutes. Turn the beef strips with kitchen tongs and cook further for 3 minutes.

2. Once ready, remove the beef to a safe-oven dish that fits in the fryer's basket. Add the rice, broccoli, green beans, garlic, ginger, sesame oil, vinegar, and soy sauce. Mix evenly using a spoon.

3. Place the dish in the fryer basket, close, and cook at 370 F for 10 minutes. Open the Air Fryer, mix the rice well, and cook for 4 minutes; season with salt and pepper. Dish the rice into serving bowls and serve with hot sauce.

Mustard Pork Chops With Lemon Zest

Preparation Time: 10 minutes

Cooking time: 25 minutes

Servings: 3

Ingredients:

- Three lean pork chops

- Salt and black pepper to taste to season

- Two eggs, cracked into a bowl

- 1tbsp water

- 1cup breadcrumbs

- ½ tsp. garlic powder

- 3 tsp. paprika

- 1½ tsp. Oregano

- ½ tsp. Cayenne pepper

- ¼ tsp. dry mustard

- One lemon, zested

Directions:

1. Put the pork chops on a chopping board and use a knife to trim off any excess fat. Add the water to the eggs and whisk; set aside. In another bowl, add the breadcrumbs, salt, pepper, garlic powder, paprika, oregano, cayenne pepper, lemon zest, and dry mustard. Use a fork to mix evenly.

2. Preheat the Air Fryer to 380 F and grease the basket with cooking spray. In the egg mixture, dip each pork chop and then in the breadcrumb mixture. Place the breaded chops in the fryer. Don't spray with cooking spray. The fat in the chops will be enough oil to cook them. Close the Air Fryer and cook for 12 minutes.

3. Flip to other side and cook for another 5 minutes.

4. Once ready, place the chops on a chopping board to rest for 3 minutes before slicing and serving. Serve with a side of vegetable fries.

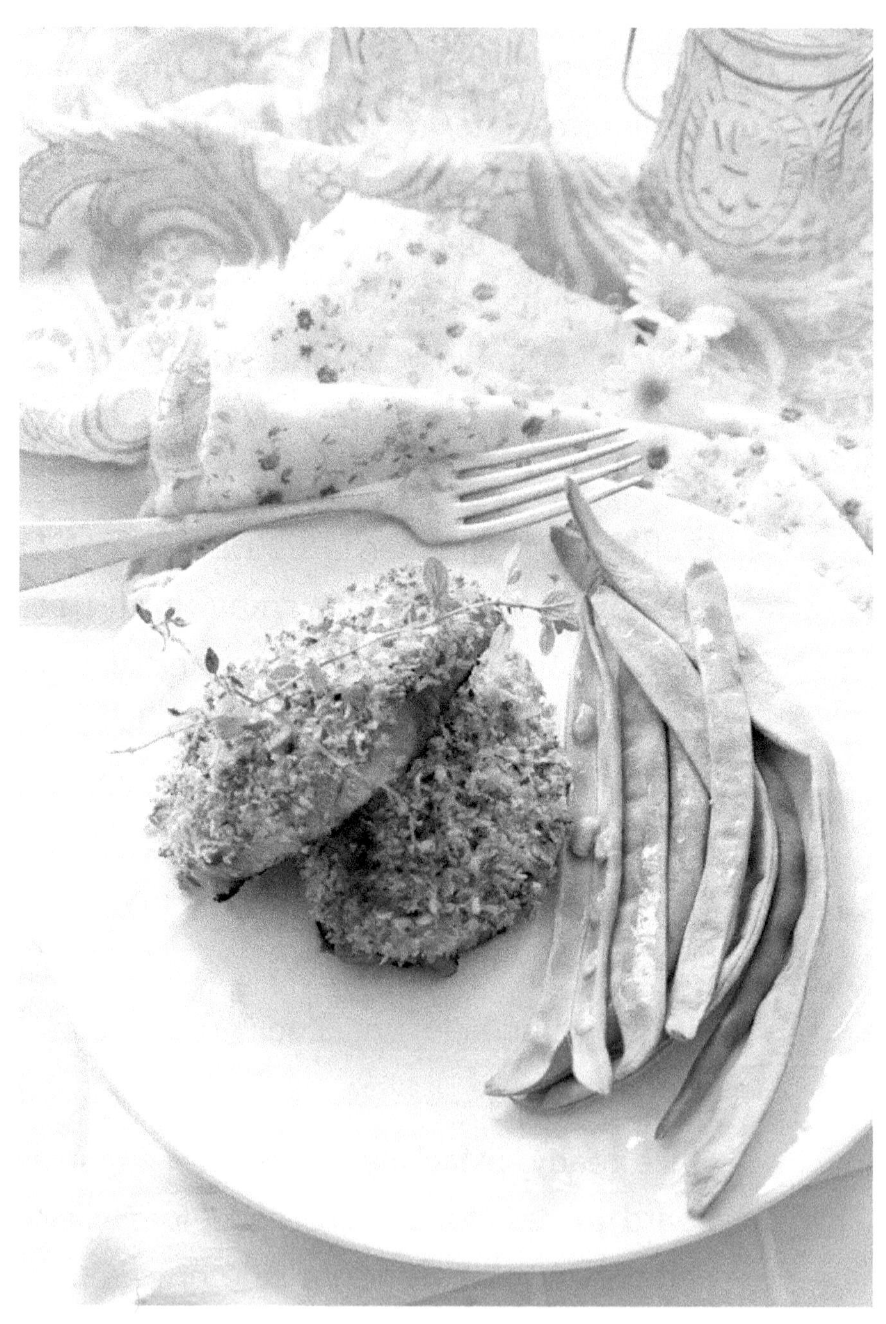

Herbed Beef Roast

Preparation Time: 10 minutes

Cooking time: 50 minutes

Servings: 2

Ingredients:

- 2 tsp. olive oil
- 1 lb. beef roast
- ½ tsp. Dried rosemary
- ½ tsp. Dried thyme
- ½ tsp. dried oregano
- Salt and black pepper to taste

Directions:

1. Preheat the Air Fryer to 400 F. Drizzle oil over the beef, and sprinkle with salt, pepper, and herbs. Rub onto the meat with hands.

2. Cook for 45 minutes for medium-rare and 50 minutes for well-done.

3. Check halfway through, and flip to ensure they cook evenly.

4. Wrap the beef in foil for 10 minutes after cooking to allow the juices to reabsorb into the meat. Slice the beef and serve with a side of steamed asparagus.

Roast Pork Belly With Cumin

Preparation: 15 minutes

Cooking time: 4 hours and 30 minutes

Servings: 8

Ingredients:

- 1½ lb. pork belly

- 1½ tsp. Garlic powder

- ½ tsp. Coriander powder

- ⅓ tsp. Salt

- ½ tsp. Black pepper

- ½ dried thyme

- ½ tsp. dried oregano

- 1½ tsp. cumin powder

- 3 cups of water

- lemon halved

Directions:

1. Leave the pork to air fry for 3 hours. In a small bowl, add the garlic powder, coriander powder, ½ tsp. of salt, black pepper, thyme, oregano, and cumin powder. After the pork is well dried, poke holes all around it using a fork. Smear the oregano, rub thoroughly on all sides with your hands, and squeeze the lemon juice all over it.

2. Leave to sit for 5 minutes. Put the pork in the center of the fryer basket and cook for 30 minutes. Turn the pork with two spatulas, increase the temperature to 350 F and continue cooking for 25 minutes.

3. Once ready, remove it and place it on a chopping board to sit for 4 minutes before slicing. Serve the pork slices with a side of sautéed asparagus and hot sauce.

Sunday Night Garlic Beef Schnitzel

Preparation Time: 8minutes

Cooking time: 22 minutes

Servings: 1

Ingredients:

- 2 tbsp. olive oil

- One thin beef cutlet

- One egg, beaten

- 2 oz. breadcrumbs

- 1tsp paprika

- ¼ tsp. garlic powder

- Salt and black pepper to taste

Directions:

1. Preheat the air fryer to 350 F. Combine olive oil, breadcrumbs, paprika, garlic powder, and salt in a bowl. Dip the beef in with the egg first, and then coat it with the breadcrumb mixture thoroughly.

2. Line a baking dish with parchment paper and place the breaded meat on it.

3. Cook for 12 minutes. Serve and enjoy.

Meatballs With Parsley And Thyme

Preparation Time: 10 minutes

Cooking time: 25 minutes

Servings: 6

Ingredients:

- One small onion, chopped
- ¾ pound grounded beef
- 1tbsp fresh parsley, chopped
- ½ tbsp. fresh thyme leaves, chopped
- whole egg, beaten
- 3 tbsp. breadcrumbs
- Salt and black pepper to taste
- Tomato sauce for coating

Directions:

1. Preheat your Air Fryer to 390 F. In a mixing bowl, mix all the Ingredients: except tomato sauce. Roll the mixture into 10-12 balls.

2. Place the balls in your air fryer's cooking basket, and cook for 8 minutes. Add tomato sauce to the balls to coat and cook for 5 minutes at 300 F.

3. Gently stir and enjoy!

Garlic Lamb Chops With Thyme

Preparation Time: 10 minutes

Cooking time: 30 minutes

Servings: 4

Ingredients:

- Four lamb chops
- One garlic clove, peeled
- 1 tbsp. plus
- 2 tsp. Olive oil
- ½ tbsp. Oregano
- ½ tbsp. Thyme
- ½ tsp. Salt
- ¼ tsp. black pepper

Directions:

1. Preheat the air fryer to 390 F. Coat the garlic clove with 1 tsp. Of olive oil and place it in the air fryer for 10 minutes. Meanwhile, mix the herbs and seasonings with the remaining olive oil.

2. Using a towel or a mitten, squeeze the hot roasted garlic clove into the herb mixture and stir to combine.

3. Coat the lamb chops with the mixture well, and place it in the air fryer—Cook for 8 to 12 minutes.

Ginger Rack Rib Steak

Preparation Time: 10 minutes

Cooking time: 35 minutes

Servings: 2

Ingredients:

- One rack rib steak
- Salt to season
- 1tsp white pepper
- 1tsp garlic powder
- ½ tsp. red pepper flakes
- 1tsp ginger powder
- 1cup Hot sauce

Directions:

1. Preheat the Air Fryer to 360 F. Place the rib rack on a flat surface and pat dry using a paper towel. Season the ribs with salt, garlic, ginger, white pepper, and red pepper flakes.

2. Place the ribs in the fryer's basket and cook for 15 minutes. Turn the ribs with kitchen

tongs and cook further for 15 minutes.

3. Remove the ribs onto a chopping board and let sit for 3 minutes before slicing. Plate and drizzle hot sauce over and serve.

Cheeseburger Egg Rolls

Preparation Time: 10 minutes

Cooking Time: 7 minutes

Serving: 6

Ingredients

- 6egg roll wrappers
- 6chopped dill pickle chips
- 1tbsp. yellow mustard
- 3tbsp. Cream cheese
- tbsp. shredded cheddar cheese
- ½ C. chopped onion
- ½ C. chopped bell pepper
- ¼ tsp. Onion powder
- ¼ tsp. garlic powder
- 8 ounces of raw lean ground beef

Directions:

1. In a skillet, add seasonings, beef, onion, and bell pepper. Stir and crumble beef till fully cooked, and vegetables are soft.

2. Take the skillet off the heat and add cream cheese, mustard, and cheddar cheese, stirring till melted.

3. Pour beef mixture into a bowl and fold in pickles.

4. Layout egg wrappers and place 1/6th of beef mixture into each one. Moisten egg roll wrapper edges with water. Fold sides to the middle and seal with water.

5. Repeat with all other egg rolls.

6. Place rolls into the air fryer, one batch at a time.

7. Pour into the Oven rack/basket. Place the Rack on the middle-shelf of the Air Fryer Oven. Set temperature to 392°F, and set time to 7 minutes.

Nutrition: CALORIES: 153; FAT: 4G; PROTEIN: 12G; SUGAR: 3G

Air Fried Grilled Steak

Preparation Time: 5 minutes

Cooking Time: 45 minutes

Serving: 2

Ingredients

- 2top sirloin steaks

- 3tablespoons butter, melted

- 3tablespoons olive oil

- Salt and pepper to taste

Directions:

1. Preheat the Air Fryer Oven for 5 minutes.

2. Season the sirloin steaks with olive oil, salt, and pepper.

3. Place the beef in the air fryer basket.

4. Cook for 45 minutes at 350°F.

5. Once cooked, serve with butter.

Nutrition: CALORIES: 1536; FAT: 123.7G; PROTEIN: 103.4G

Juicy Cheeseburgers

Preparation Time: 5 minutes

Cooking Time: 15 minutes

Serving: 4

Ingredients

- 1pound 93% lean ground beef

- 1teaspoon Worcestershire sauce

- 1tablespoon burger seasoning

- Salt

- Pepper

- Cooking oil

- 4slices cheese

- buns

Directions:

1. In a large bowl, mix the ground beef, Worcestershire, burger seasoning, salt, and pepper to taste until well blended. Spray the air fryer basket with cooking oil. You will need only a quick spritz. The burgers will produce oil as they cook.

Shape the mixture into four patties. Place the burgers in the air fryer. The burgers should fit without the need to stack, but stacking is okay if necessary.

2. Pour into the Oven rack/basket. Place the Rack on the middle-shelf of the Casoria Air Fryer Oven. Set temperature to 375°F, and set time to 8 minutes. Cook for 8 minutes. Open the air fryer and flip the burgers— Cook for an additional 3 to 4 minutes. Check the inside of the burgers to determine if they have finished cooking. You can stick a knife or fork in the center to examine the color.

3. Top each burger with a slice of cheese— Cook for an additional minute, or until the cheese has melted. Serve on buns with any different toppings of your choice.

Nutrition: CALORIES: 566; FAT: 39G; PROTEIN: 29G; FIBER: 1G

Spicy Thai Beef Stir-Fry

Preparation Time: 15 minutes

Cooking Time: 9 minutes

Serving: 4

Ingredients

- 1pound sirloin steaks, thinly sliced

- 2tablespoons lime juice, divided

- ⅓ cup crunchy peanut butter

- ½ cup beef broth

- 1tablespoon olive oil

- 1½ cups broccoli florets

- 2cloves garlic, sliced

- 1to 2 red Chile peppers, sliced

Directions:

1. In a medium bowl, combine the steak with one tablespoon of the lime juice. Set aside.

2. Combine the peanut butter and beef broth in a small bowl and mix well. Drain the beef and add the juice from the bowl into the peanut butter mixture.

3. In a 6-inch metal bowl, combine the olive oil, steak, and broccoli.

4. Pour into the Oven rack/basket. Place the Rack on the middle-shelf of the Air Fryer Oven. Set temperature to 375°F, and set time to 4 minutes. Cook for 3 to 4 minutes or until the steak is almost cooked and the broccoli is crisp and tender, shaking the basket once during cooking time.

5. Add the garlic, Chile peppers, and the peanut butter mixture and stir.

6. Cook for 3 to 5 minutes or until the sauce is bubbling, and the broccoli is tender.

7. Serve over hot rice.

Nutrition: CALORIES: 387; FAT: 22G; PROTEIN: 42G; FIBER: 2G

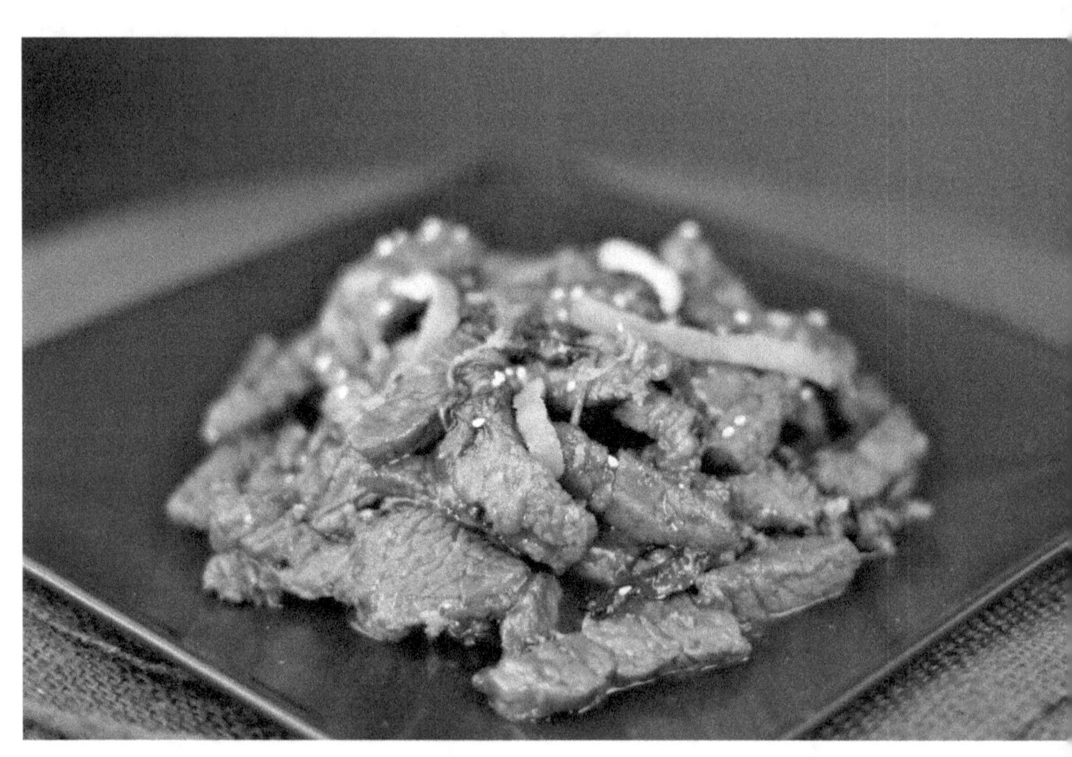

Beef Brisket Recipe From Texas

Preparation Time: 15 minutes

Cooking Time: 90 minutes

Serving: 8

Ingredients:

- ½ cup beef stock
- 1bay leaf
- 1tablespoon garlic powder
- 1tablespoon onion powder
- 2pounds beef brisket, trimmed
- 2tablespoons chili powder
- 2teaspoons dry mustard
- 4tablespoons olive oil
- Salt and pepper to taste

Directions:

1. Preheat the Air Fryer Oven for 5 minutes. Place all ingredients in a deep baking dish that will fit in the air fryer.

2. Bake for 1 hour and 30 minutes at 400°F.

3. Stir the beef after every 30 minutes to soak in the sauce.

Nutrition: CALORIES: 306; FAT: 24.1G; PROTEIN: 18.3G

Copycat Taco Bell Crunch Wraps

Preparation Time: 10 minutes

Cooking Time: 2 minutes

Serving: 6

Ingredients

- 6wheat tostadas
- 2C. sour cream
- 2C. Mexican blend cheese
- 2C. shredded lettuce
- 12 ounces low-sodium nacho cheese
- Roma t3omatoes
- 6-12-inch wheat tortillas
- 1 1/3 C. water
- 2packets low-sodium taco seasoning
- 2pounds of lean ground beef

Directions:

1. Ensure your air fryer is preheated to 400 degrees.

2. Make beef according to taco seasoning packets.

3. Place 2/3 C. prepared beef, 4 tbsp. Cheese, one tostada, 1/3 C. sour cream, 1/3 C. lettuce, 1/6th of tomatoes, and 1/3 C. cheese on each tortilla.

4. Fold up tortillas edges and repeat with remaining ingredients.

5. Lay the folded sides of tortillas down into the air fryer and spray with olive oil.

6. Set temperature to 400°F, and set time to 2 minutes. Cook 2 minutes till browned.

Nutrition: CALORIES: 311; FAT: 9G; PROTEIN: 22G; SUGAR: 2G

Air Fryer Beef Casserole

Preparation Time: 5 minutes

Cooking Time: 30 minutes

Serving: 4

Ingredients

- One green bell pepper, seeded and chopped
- One onion, chopped
- 1-pound ground beef
- 3cloves of garlic, minced
- 3tablespoons olive oil
- 6cups eggs, beaten
- Salt and pepper to taste

Directions:

1. Preheat the Air Fryer Oven for 5 minutes.
2. A baking dish that will fit in the air fryer, mix the ground beef, onion, garlic, olive oil, and bell pepper—season with salt and pepper to taste.

3. Pour in the beaten eggs and give a good stir.

4. Place the dish with the beef and egg mixture in the air fryer.

5. Pour into the Oven rack/basket. Place the Rack on the middle-shelf of the Air Fryer Oven. Set temperature to 325°F, and set time to 30 minutes. Bake for 30 minutes.

Nutrition: CALORIES: 1520; FAT: 125.11G; PROTEIN: 87.9G

Meat Lovers' Pizza

Preparation Time: 10 minutes

Cooking Time: 12 minutes

Serving: 2

Ingredients

- 1pre-prepared 7-inch pizza crust, defrosted if necessary.

- 1/3 cup of marinara sauce.

- 2ounces of grilled steak, sliced into bite-sized pieces

- 2ounces of salami, cut fine

- 2ounces of pepperoni, cut fine

- ¼ cup of American cheese

- ¼ cup of shredded mozzarella cheese

Directions:

1. Preheat the Air Fryer Oven to 350 degrees. Lay the pizza dough flat on a sheet of parchment paper or tin foil, cut large enough to hold the entire pie crust but small enough that it will leave the edges of the air frying basket uncovered to allow for

air circulation.

2. Using a fork, stab the pizza dough several times across the surface – piercing the pie crust will allow air to circulate throughout the crust and ensure even cooking. With a deep soup spoon, scoop the marinara sauce onto the pizza dough, and spread evenly in expanding circles over the pie-crust surface.

3. Be sure to leave at least ½ inch of bare dough around the edges to ensure that extra-crispy crunchy first bite of the crust! Distribute the steak pieces and the slices of salami and pepperoni evenly over the sauce-covered dough, then sprinkle the cheese in an even layer on top.

4. Set the air fryer timer to 12 minutes, and place the pizza with foil or paper on the fryer's basket surface. Again, be sure to leave the edges of the basket uncovered to allow for proper air circulation, and don't let your bare fingers touch the hot surface. After 12 minutes, when the Air Fryer Oven

shuts off, the cheese should be perfectly melted and lightly crisped, and the pie crust should be golden brown. If necessary, using a spatula – or two, remove the pizza from the air fryer basket and set on a serving plate. Wait a few minutes until the pie is cool enough to handle, then cut into slices and serve.

Chimichurri Skirt Steak

Preparation Time: 10 minutes

Cooking Time: 8 minutes

Serving: 2

Ingredients

- 2x 8 oz. Skirt Steak
- 1cup Finely Chopped Parsley
- ¼ cup Finely Chopped Mint
- 2Tbsp Fresh Oregano (Washed & finely chopped)
- 3Finely Chopped Cloves of Garlic
- 1Tsp Red Pepper Flakes (Crushed)
- 1Tbsp Ground Cumin
- 1Tsp Cayenne Pepper
- 2Tsp Smoked Paprika
- 1Tsp Salt
- ¼ Tsp. Pepper
- ¾ cup Oil
- 3Tbsp Red Wine Vinegar

Directions:

1. Throw all the ingredients in a bowl (besides the steak) and mix well.

2. Put ¼ cup of the mixture in a plastic baggie with the steak and leave in the fridge overnight (2–24hrs).

3. Leave the bag out at room temperature for at least 30 min before popping into the air fryer. Preheat for a minute or two to 390° F before cooking until med–rare (8–10 min). Pour into the Oven rack/basket. Place the Rack on the middle-shelf of the Air Fryer Oven. Set temperature to 390°F, and set time to 10 minutes.

4. Put 2 Tbsp. Of the chimichurri, mix on top of each steak before serving.

Country Fried Steak

Preparation Time: 5 minutes

Cooking Time: 12 minutes

Serving: 2

Ingredients

- 1tsp. pepper

- 2C. almond milk

- 2tbsp. almond flour

- 6ounces ground sausage meat

- 1tsp. pepper

- 1tsp. salt

- 1tsp. garlic powder

- 1tsp. onion powder

- 1C. panko breadcrumbs

- 1C. almond flour

- 3beaten eggs

- 6ounces sirloin steak pounded till thin

Directions:

1. Season panko breadcrumbs with spices.

2. Dredge steak in flour, then egg, and then seasoned panko mixture.

3. Place into an air fryer basket.

4. Set temperature to 370°F, and set time to 12 minutes.

5. To make sausage gravy, cook sausage and drain off fat, but reserve two tablespoons.

6. Add flour to sausage and mix until incorporated. Gradually mix in milk over medium to high heat till it becomes thick.

7. Season mixture with pepper and cook 3 minutes longer.

8. Serve steak topped with gravy and enjoy.

Nutrition: CALORIES: 395; FAT: 11G; PROTEIN: 39G; SUGAR: 5G

Italian Meatballs

Preparation Time: 15 minutes

Cooking Time: 25 minutes

Serving: 4

Ingredients:

- 1pound ground beef (80% lean)

- ⅓ cup breadcrumbs

- ¼ cup milk

- 2eggs

- 2teaspoons garlic powder

- 1teaspoon onion powder

- ½ teaspoon red chili flakes

- 3teaspoons dried oregano

- 2tablespoons fresh parsley, chopped

- ¼ cup Parmesan cheese, grated

- Salt & pepper, to taste

Directions:

1. Combine all ingredients in a large bowl. Mix well.

2. Roll the mixture into medium-sized balls. Chill in the fridge for 10 minutes.

3. Select the Air Fry function on the COSORI Air Fryer Toaster Oven and press Start/Cancel to preheat.

4. Line the fry basket with parchment paper, and then place the meatballs in the basket.

5. Insert the fry basket at mid-position in the preheated air fryer toaster oven. Press Start/Cancel.

6. Remove when done and then serve.

Nutrition:

Calories 316, Total Fat 12g, Carbs 10g, Protein 42g

Lamb Chops With Rosemary Sauce

Prep Time: 10 minutes

Cooking Time: 52 minutes

Serving: 8

Ingredients

- Eight lamb loin chops

- One small onion, peeled and chopped

- Salt and black pepper, to taste

For the sauce:

- One onion, peeled and chopped

- One tablespoon rosemary leaves

- 1 oz. butter

- 1 oz. plain flour

- Six fly oz. milk

- Six fly oz. vegetable stock

- • Two tablespoons cream, whipping

- • Salt and black pepper, to taste

Directions:

1. Place the lamb loin chops and onion in a baking tray, and then drizzle salt and black pepper on top.

2. Press "Power Button" of Air Fry Oven and turn the dial to select the "Bake" mode.

3. Press the Time button and again turn the dial to set the cooking time to 45 minutes.

4. Now push the Temp button and rotate the dial to set the temperature at 350 degrees F.

5. Once preheated, place the lamb baking tray in the oven and close its lid.

6. Prepare the white sauce by melting butter in a saucepan, and then stir in onions.

7. Sauté for 5 minutes, then stir flour and stir cook for 2 minutes.

8. Stir in the rest of the ingredients and mix well.

9. Pour the sauce over baked chops and serve.

Nutrition:

Calories 284

Total Fat 7.9 g

Saturated Fat 1.4 g

Cholesterol 36 mg

Sodium 704 mg

Total Carbs 46 g

Fiber 3.6 g

Sugar 5.5 g

Protein 17.9 g

Roast Lamb Shoulder

Prep Time: 10 minutes

Cooking Time: 60 minutes

Serving: 2

Ingredients

- 1 lb. boneless lamb shoulder roast

- Four cloves garlic, minced

- One tablespoon rosemary, chopped

- Two teaspoon thyme leaves

- Three tablespoon olive oil, divided

- **Salt**

- Black pepper

- 2 lb. baby potatoes halved

Directions:

- Toss potatoes with all the herbs, seasonings, and oil in a baking tray.

- Press "Power Button" of Air Fry Oven and turn the dial to select the "Air

Roast" mode.

• Press the Time button and again turn the dial to set the cooking time to 60 minutes.

• Now push the Temp button and rotate the dial to set the temperature at 370 degrees F.

• Once preheated, place the lamb baking tray in the oven and close its lid.

• Slice and serve warm.

Nutrition:

Calories 134

Total Fat 4.7 g

Saturated Fat 0.6 g

Cholesterol 124mg

Sodium 1 mg

Total Carbs 54.1 g

Fiber 7 g

Sugar 3.3 g

Protein 26.2 g

Garlicky Lamb Chops

Prep Time: 10 minutes

Cooking Time: 45 minutes

Serving: 8

Ingredients

- Eight medium lamb chops
- 1/4 cup olive oil
- Three thin lemon slices
- Two garlic cloves, crushed
- One teaspoon dried oregano
- One teaspoon salt
- 1/2 teaspoon black pepper

Directions:

1. Place the medium lamb chops in a baking tray and rub them with olive oil.

2. Add lemon slices, garlic, oregano, salt, and black pepper on top of the lamb chops.

3. Press "Power Button" of Air Fry Oven and turn the dial to select the "Air Roast" mode.

4. Press the Time button and again turn the dial to set the cooking time to 45 minutes.

5. Now push the Temp button and rotate the dial to set the temperature at 400 degrees F.

6. Once preheated, place the lamb baking tray in the oven and close its lid.

7. Slice and serve warm.

Nutrition:

Calories 387

Total Fat 6 g

Saturated Fat 9.9 g

Cholesterol 41 mg

Sodium 154 mg

Total Carbs 37.4 g

Fiber 2.9 g

Sugar 15.3 g

Protein 14.6 g

New England Lamb

Prep Time: 10 minutes

Cooking Time: 60 minutes

Serving: 6

Ingredients

- Two tablespoon canola oil

- 2 lbs. boneless leg of lamb, diced

- One onion, chopped

- Two leeks white portion only, sliced

- Two carrots, sliced

- Two tablespoons minced fresh parsley, divided

- 1/2 teaspoon dried rosemary, crushed

- 1/2 teaspoon salt

- 1/4 teaspoon black pepper

- 1/4 teaspoon dried thyme, crushed

- Three potatoes, peeled and sliced

- Three tablespoons butter, melted

Directions:

1. Toss the lamb cubes with all the veggies, oil, and seasonings in a baking tray.

2. Press "Power Button" of Air Fry Oven and turn the dial to select the "Air Roast" mode.

3. Press the Time button and again turn the dial to set the cooking time to 60 minutes.

4. Now push the Temp button and rotate the dial to set the temperature at 350 degrees F.

5. Once preheated, place the lamb baking tray in the oven and close its lid.

6. Slice and serve warm.

Nutrition:

Calories 212

Total Fat 11.8 g

Saturated Fat 2.2 g

Cholesterol 23mg

Sodium 321 mg

Total Carbs 14.6 g

Dietary Fiber 4.4 g

Sugar 8 g

Protein 17.3 g

Onion Lamb Kebabs

Prep Time: 10 minutes

Cooking Time: 20 minutes

Serving: 4

Ingredients

- 18 oz. lamb kebab
- One teaspoon chili powder
- One teaspoon cumin powder
- One egg
- 2 oz. onion, chopped
- Two teaspoon sesame oil

Directions:

1. Whisk onion with egg, chili powder, oil, cumin powder, and salt in a bowl.

2. Add lamb to coat well, and then thread it on the skewers.

3. Place these lamb skewers in the Air fryer basket.

4. Press "Power Button" of Air Fry Oven and turn the dial to select the "Air Fry" mode.

5. Press the Time button and again turn the dial to set the cooking time to 20 minutes.

6. Now push the Temp button and rotate the dial to set the temperature at 395 degrees F.

7. Once preheated, place the Air fryer basket in the oven and close its lid.

8. Slice and serve warm.

Nutrition:

Calories 412

Total Fat 24.8 g

Saturated Fat 12.4 g

Cholesterol 3 mg

Sodium 132 mg

Total Carbs 43.8 g

Dietary Fiber 3.9 g

Sugar 2.5 g

Protein 18.9 g

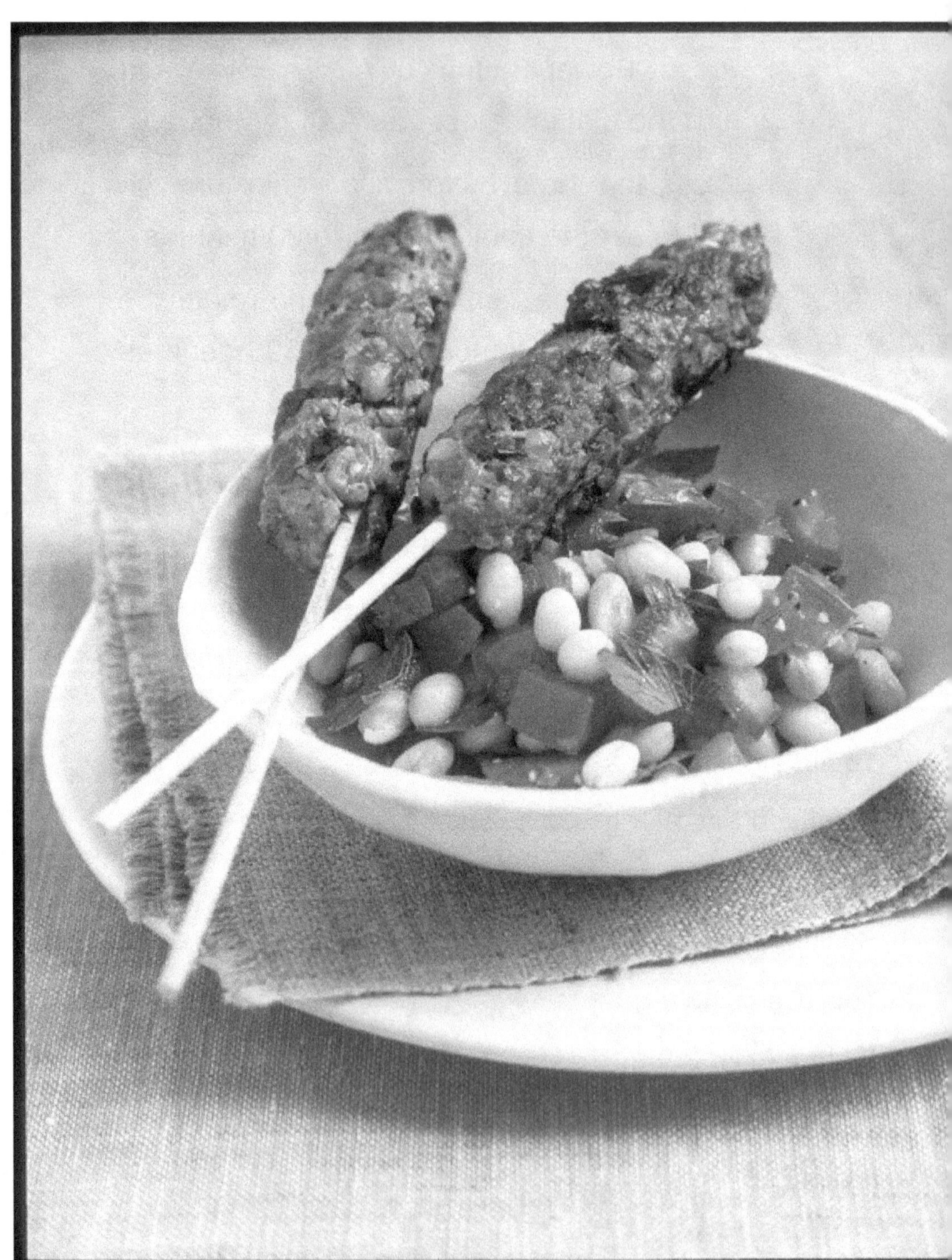

Zucchini Lamb Meatballs

Prep Time: 10 minutes

Cooking Time: 15 minutes

Serving: 4

Ingredients

- 1 lb. ground lamb

- avocado oil spray

- 1/2 tablespoon garlic ghee

- One red bell pepper diced

- 1/3 cup red onion diced

- 1/3 cup cilantro diced

- 1/3 cup zucchini diced

- One tablespoon gyro seasoning

- 1/2 teaspoon turmeric

- 1/2 teaspoon cumin

- 1/2 teaspoon coriander

- Two garlic cloves minced

- Salt and black pepper to taste

Directions:

1. Mix the lamb minced with all the meatball ingredients in a bowl.

2. Make small meatballs out of this mixture and place them in the air fryer basket.

3. Press "Power Button" of Air Fry Oven and turn the dial to select the "Air Fry" mode.

4. Press the Time button and again turn the dial to set the cooking time to 15 minutes.

5. Now push the Temp button and rotate the dial to set the temperature at 370 degrees F.

6. Once preheated, place the Air fryer basket in the oven and close its lid.

7. Slice and serve warm.

Nutrition:

Calories 331

Total Fat 2.5 g

Saturated Fat 0.5 g

Cholesterol 35 mg

Sodium 595 mg

Total Carbs 69 g

Fiber 12.2 g

Sugar 12.5 g

Protein 8.7g

Mint Lamb With Roasted Hazelnuts

Prep Time: 10 minutes

Cooking Time: 25 minutes

Serving: 2

Ingredients

- ¼ cup hazelnuts, toasted

- 2/3 lb. shoulder of lamb cut into strips

- One tablespoon hazelnut oil

- Two tablespoons fresh mint leaves chopped

- ½ cup frozen peas

- ¼ cup of water

- ½ cup white wine

- Salt and black pepper to taste

Directions:

1. Toss lamb with hazelnuts, spices, and all the ingredients in a baking pan.

2. Press "Power Button" of Air Fry Oven and turn the dial to select the "Bake" mode.

3. Press the Time button and again turn the dial to set the cooking time to 25 minutes.

4. Now push the Temp button and rotate the dial to set the temperature at 370 degrees F.

5. Once preheated, place the baking pan in the oven and close its lid.

6. Slice and serve warm.

Nutrition:

Calories 322

Total Fat 11.8 g

Saturated Fat 2.2 g

Cholesterol 56 mg

Sodium 321 mg

Total Carbs 14.6 g

Dietary Fiber 4.4 g

Sugar 8 g

Protein 19.3 g

Lamb Rack With Lemon Crust

Prep Time: 10 minutes

Cooking Time: 25 minutes

Serving: 5

Ingredients

- 1.7 lbs. frenched rack of lamb
- Salt and black pepper, to taste
- 0.13-lb. dry breadcrumbs
- One teaspoon grated garlic
- 1/2 teaspoon salt
- One teaspoon cumin seeds
- One teaspoon ground cumin
- One teaspoon oil
- ½ teaspoon Grated lemon rind
- One egg, beaten

Directions:

1. Place the lamb rack in a baking tray and pour the whisked egg on top.

2. Whisk the rest of the crusting ingredients in a bowl and spread over the lamb.

3. Press "Power Button" of Air Fry Oven and turn the dial to select the "Air Fry" mode.

4. Press the Time button and again turn the dial to set the cooking time to 25 minutes.

5. Now push the Temp button and rotate the dial to set the temperature at 350 degrees F.

6. Once preheated, place the lamb baking tray in the oven and close its lid.

7. Slice and serve warm.

Nutrition:

Calories 427

Total Fat 5.4 g

Saturated Fat 4.2 g

Cholesterol 168 mg

Sodium 203 mg

Total Carbs 58.5 g

Sugar 1.1 g

Fiber 4 g

Protein 21.9 g

Braised Lamb Shanks

Prep Time: 10 minutes

Cooking Time: 20 minutes

Serving: 4

Ingredients

- Four lamb shanks
- 1½ teaspoons salt
- ½ teaspoon black pepper
- Four garlic cloves, crushed
- Two tablespoons olive oil
- 4 to 6 sprigs fresh rosemary
- 3 cups beef broth, divided
- Two tablespoons balsamic vinegar

Directions:

1. Place the sham shanks in a baking pan.

2. Whisk the rest of the ingredients in a bowl and pour over the shanks.

3. Place these shanks in the Air fryer basket.

4. Press "Power Button" of Air Fry Oven and turn the dial to select the "Air Fry" mode.

5. Press the Time button and again turn the dial to set the cooking time to 20 minutes.

6. Now push the Temp button and rotate the dial to set the temperature at 360 degrees F.

7. Once preheated, place the Air fryer basket in the oven and close its lid.

8. Slice and serve warm.

Nutrition:

Calories 336

Total Fat 9.7 g

Saturated Fat 4.7 g

Cholesterol 181 mg

Sodium 245 mg

Total Carbs 32.5 g

Fiber 0.3 g

Sugar 1.8 g

Protein 30.3 g

Za'atar Lamb Chops

Prep Time: 10 minutes

Cooking Time: 10 minutes

Serving: 8

Ingredients

- Eight lamb loin chops, bone-in
- Three garlic cloves, crushed
- One teaspoon olive oil
- 1/2 fresh lemon
- 1 1/4 teaspoon salt
- One tablespoon Za'atar
- Black pepper, to taste

Directions:

1. Rub the lamb chops with oil, zaatar, salt, lemon juice, garlic, and black pepper.

2. Place these chops in the air fryer basket.

3. Press "Power Button" of Air Fry Oven and turn the dial to select the "Air Fry" mode.

4. Press the Time button and again turn the dial to set the cooking time to 10 minutes.

5. Now push the Temp button and rotate the dial to set the temperature at 400 degrees F.

6. Once preheated, place the air fryer basket in the oven and close its lid.

7. Flip the chops when cooked halfway through, and then resume cooking.

8. Serve warm.

Nutrition:

Calories 391

Total Fat 2.8 g

Saturated Fat 0.6 g

Cholesterol 330 mg

Sodium 62 mg

Total Carbs 36.5 g

Fiber 9.2 g

Sugar 4.5 g

Protein 6.6

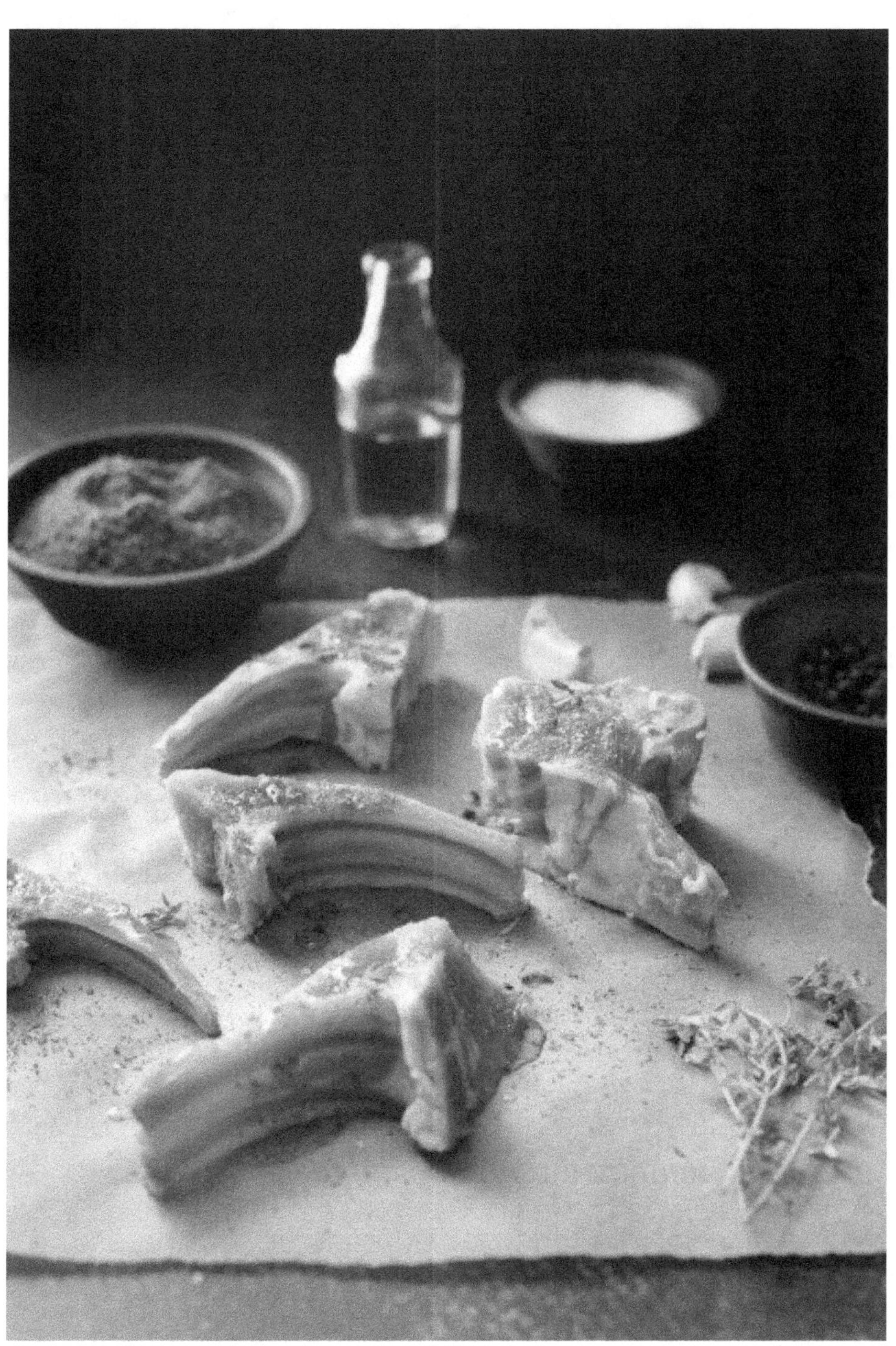

Simple Beef Sirloin Roast

Preparation Time: 10 minutes

Cooking Time: 50 minutes

Servings: 8

Ingredients:

- 2½ pounds sirloin roast
- Salt and ground black pepper, as required

Directions:

1. Rub the roast with salt and black pepper generously.

2. Insert the rotisserie rod through the roast.

3. Insert the rotisserie forks, one on each rod's side, to secure the rod to the chicken.

4. Arrange the drip pan at the bottom of the Instant Vortex plus Air Fryer Oven cooking chamber.

5. Select "Roast" and then adjust the temperature to 350 degrees F.

6. Set the timer for 50 minutes and press the "Start."

7. When the display shows "Add Food," press the red lever down and load the rod's left side into the Vortex.

8. Now, slide the rod's left side into the groove along the metal bar, so it doesn't move.

9. Then, close the door and touch "Rotate."

10. When cooking time is complete, press the red lever to release the rod.

11. Remove from the Vortex and place the roast onto a platter for about 10 minutes before slicing.

12. With a sharp knife, cut the roast into desired sized slices and serve.

Nutrition:

Calories 201

Total Fat 8.8 g

Saturated Fat 3.1 g

Cholesterol 94 mg

Sodium 88 mg

Total Carbs 0 g

Fiber 0 g

Sugar 0 g

Protein 28.9 g

Seasoned Beef Roast

Preparation Time: 10 minutes

Cooking Time: 45 minutes

Servings: 10

Ingredients:

- 3 pounds beef top roast
- One tablespoon olive oil
- Two tablespoons Montreal steak seasoning

Directions:

1. Coat the roast with oil and then rub with the seasoning generously.

2. With kitchen twines, tie the roast to keep it compact.

3. Arrange the roast onto the cooking tray.

4. Arrange the drip pan at the bottom of the Instant Vortex plus Air Fryer Oven cooking chamber.

5. Select "Air Dry" and then adjust the temperature to 360 degrees F.

6. Set the timer for 45 minutes and press the "Start."

7. When the display shows "Add Food," insert the cooking tray in the center position.

8. When the display shows "Turn Food," do nothing.

9. When cooking time is complete, remove the tray from Vortex and place the roast onto a platter for about 10 minutes before slicing.

10. With a sharp knife, cut the roast into desired sized slices and serve.

Nutrition:

Calories 269

Total Fat 9.9 g

Saturated Fat 3.4 g

Cholesterol 122 mg

Sodium 538 mg

Total Carbs 0 g

Fiber 0 g

Sugar 0 g

Protein 41.3 g

Bacon-Wrapped Filet Mignon

Preparation Time: 10 minutes

Cooking Time: 15 minutes

Servings: 2

Ingredients:

- Two bacon slices

- 2 (4-ounce) filet mignon

- Salt and ground black pepper, as required

- Olive oil cooking spray

Directions:

1. Wrap 1 bacon slice around each filet mignon and secure with toothpicks.

2. Season the fillets with the salt and black pepper lightly.

3. Arrange the filet mignon onto a cooling rack and spray with cooking spray.

4. Arrange the drip pan at the bottom of the Instant Vortex plus Air Fryer Oven cooking chamber.

5. Select "Air Dry" and then adjust the temperature to 375 degrees F.

6. Set the timer for 15 minutes and press the "Start."

7. When the display shows "Add Food," insert the cooking rack in the center position.

8. When the display shows "Turn Food," turn the filets.

9. When cooking time is complete, remove the rack from Vortex and serve hot.

Nutrition:

Calories 360

Total Fat 19.6 g

Saturated Fat 6.8 g

Cholesterol 108 mg

Sodium 737 mg

Total Carbs 0.4 g

Fiber 0 g

Sugar 0 g

Protein 42.6 g

Beef Burgers

Preparation Time: 15 minutes

Cooking Time: 18 minutes

Servings: 4

Ingredients:

For Burgers:

- 1 pound ground beef

- ½ cup panko breadcrumbs

- ¼ cup onion, chopped finely

- Three tablespoons Dijon mustard

- Three teaspoons low-sodium soy sauce

- Two teaspoons fresh rosemary, chopped finely

- Salt, to taste

For Topping:

- Two tablespoons Dijon mustard

- One tablespoon brown sugar

- One teaspoon soy sauce

- 4 Gruyere cheese slices

Directions:

1. In a large bowl, add all the ingredients and mix until well combined.

2. Make four equal-sized patties from the mixture.

3. Arrange the patties onto a cooking tray.

4. Arrange the drip pan at the bottom of the Instant Vortex plus Air Fryer Oven cooking chamber.

5. Select "Air Dry" and then adjust the temperature to 370 degrees F.

6. Set the timer for 15 minutes and press the "Start."

7. When the display shows "Add Food," insert the cooking rack in the center position.

8. When the display shows "Turn Food," turn the burgers.

9. Meanwhile, for the sauce: In a small bowl, add the mustard, brown sugar, and soy sauce and mix well.

10. When cooking time is complete, remove the tray from Vortex and coat the burgers with the sauce.

11. Top each burger with one cheese slice.

12. Return the tray to the cooking chamber and select "Broil."

13. Set the timer for 3 minutes and press the "Start."

14. When cooking time is complete, remove the tray from Vortex and serve hot.

Nutrition:

Calories 402

Total Fat 18 g

Saturated Fat 8.5 g

Cholesterol 133mg

Sodium 651 mg

Total Carbs 6.3 g

Fiber 0.8 g

Sugar 3 g

Protein 44.4 g

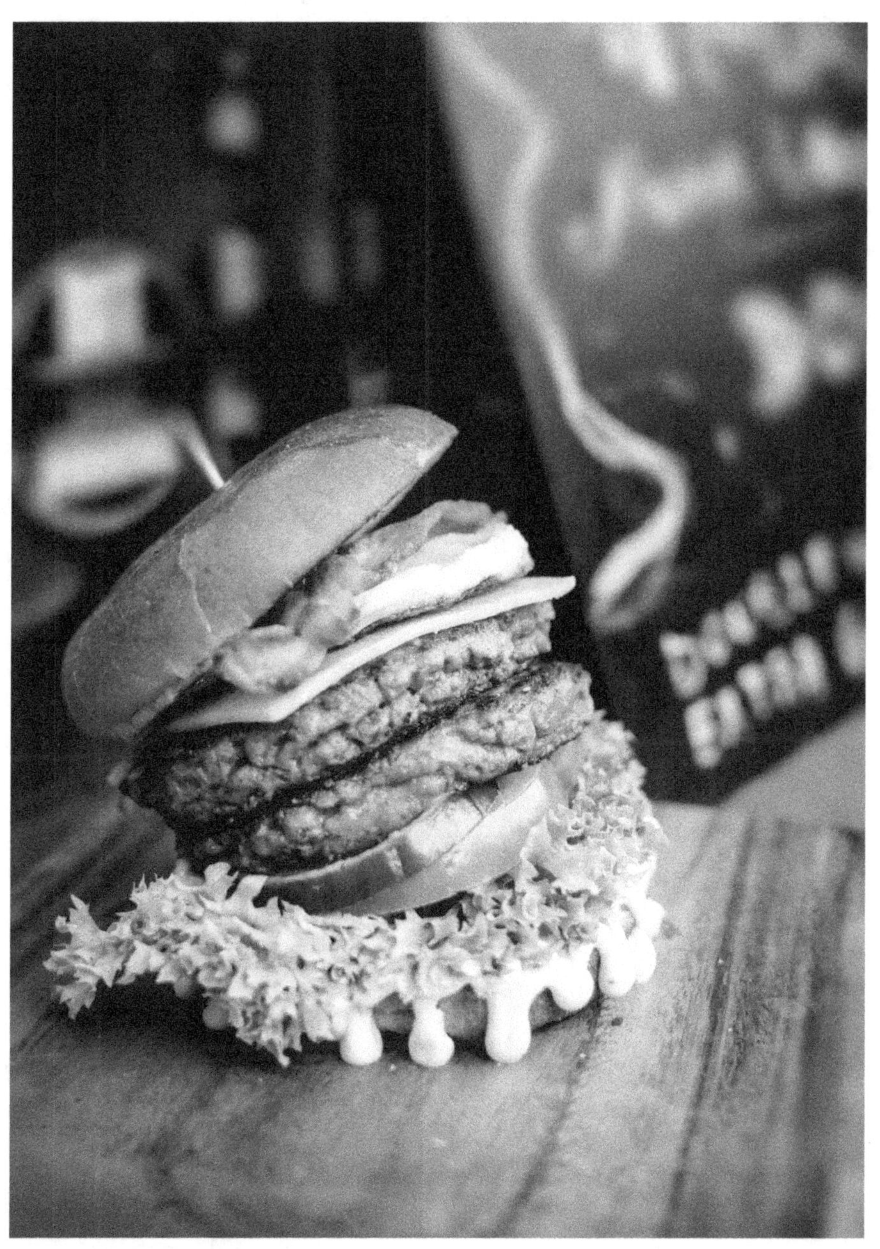

Beef Jerky

Preparation Time: 15 minutes

Cooking Time: 3 hours

Servings: 4

Ingredients:

- 1½ pounds beef round, trimmed
- ½ cup Worcestershire sauce
- ½ cup low-sodium soy sauce
- Two teaspoons honey
- One teaspoon liquid smoke
- Two teaspoons onion powder
- ½ teaspoon red pepper flakes
- Ground black pepper, as required

Directions:

1. In a zip-top bag, place the beef and freeze for 1-2 hours to firm up.

2. Place the meat onto a cutting board and cut against the grain into 1/8-¼-inch

strips.

3. In a large bowl, add the remaining ingredients and mix until well combined.

4. Add the steak slices and coat with the mixture generously.

5. Refrigerate to marinate for about 4-6 hours.

6. Remove the beef slices from the bowl, and with paper towels, pat dries them.

7. Divide the steak strips onto the cooking trays and arrange them in an even layer.

8. Select "Dehydrate" and then adjust the temperature to 160 degrees F.

9. Set the timer for 3 hours and press the "Start."

10. The display shows "Add Food" insert one tray in the top position and another in the center position.

11. After 1½ hours, switch the position of cooking trays.

12.   Meanwhile, in a small pan, add the remaining ingredients over medium heat and cook for about 10 minutes, stirring occasionally.

13.   When cooking time is complete, remove the trays from Vortex.

Nutrition:

Calories 372

Total Fat 10.7 g

Saturated Fat 4 g

Cholesterol 152 mg

Sodium 2000 mg

Total Carbs 12 g

Fiber 0.2 g

Sugar 11.3 g

Protein 53.8 g

Sweet & Spicy Meatballs

Preparation Time: 20 minutes

Cooking Time: 30 minutes

Servings: 8

Ingredients:

For Meatballs:

- 2 pounds lean ground beef
- 2/3 cup quick-cooking oats
- ½ cup Ritz crackers, crushed
- 1 (5-ounce) can evaporate milk
- Two large eggs, beaten lightly
- One teaspoon honey
- One tablespoon dried onion, minced
- One teaspoon garlic powder
- One teaspoon ground cumin
- Salt and ground black pepper, as required

For Sauce:

- 1/3 cup orange marmalade

- 1/3 cup honey

- 1/3 cup brown sugar

- Two tablespoons cornstarch

- Two tablespoons soy sauce

- 1-2 tablespoons hot sauce

- One tablespoon Worcestershire sauce

Directions:

1. For meatballs: in a large bowl, add all the ingredients and mix until well combined.

2. Make 1½-inch balls from the mixture.

3. Arrange half of the meatballs onto a cooking tray in a single layer.

4. Arrange the drip pan at the bottom of the Air Fryer Oven cooking chamber.

5. Select "Air Dry" and then adjust the temperature to 380 degrees F.

6. Set the timer for 15 minutes and press the "Start."

7. When the display shows "Add Food," insert the cooking tray in the center position.

8. When the display shows "Turn Food," turn the meatballs.

9. When cooking time is complete, remove the tray from Vortex.

10.   Repeat with the remaining meatballs.

11.   Meanwhile, for the sauce: In a small pan, add all the ingredients over medium heat and cook until thickened, stirring continuously.

12.   . Serve the meatballs with the topping of sauce.

Nutrition:

Calories 411

Total Fat 11.1 g

Saturated Fat 4.1 g

Cholesterol 153 mg

Sodium 448 mg

Total Carbs 38.8 g

Fiber 1 g

Sugar 28.1 g

Protein 38.9 g

Spiced Pork Shoulder

Preparation Time: 15 minutes

Cooking Time: 55 minutes

Servings: 6

Ingredients:

- One teaspoon ground cumin

- One teaspoon cayenne pepper

- One teaspoon garlic powder

- Salt and ground black pepper, as required

- 2 pounds skin-on pork shoulder

Directions:

1. In a small bowl, mix the spices, salt, and black pepper.

2. Arrange the pork shoulder onto a cutting board, skin-side down.

3. Season the inner side of pork shoulder with salt and black pepper.

4. With kitchen twines, tie the pork shoulder into a long round cylinder shape.

5. Season the outer side of pork shoulder with spice mixture.

6. Insert the rotisserie rod through the pork shoulder.

7. Insert the rotisserie forks, one on each side of the rod, to secure the pork shoulder.

8. Arrange the drip pan at the bottom of the Air Fryer Oven cooking chamber.

9. Select "Roast" and then adjust the temperature to 350 degrees F.

10. Set the timer for 55 minutes and press the "Start."

11. When the display shows "Add Food," press the red lever down and load the rod's left side into the Vortex.

12. Now, slide the rod's left side into the groove along the metal bar, so it doesn't move.

13. Then, close the door and touch "Rotate."

14. When cooking time is complete, press the red lever to release the rod.

15. Remove the pork from Vortex and place it onto a platter for about 10 minutes before slicing.

16. With a sharp knife, cut the pork shoulder into desired sized slices and serve.

Nutrition:

Calories 445

Total Fat 32.5 g

Saturated Fat 11.9 g

Cholesterol 136 mg

Sodium 131 mg

Total Carbs 0.7 g

Fiber 0.2 g

Sugar 0.2 g

Protein 35.4 g

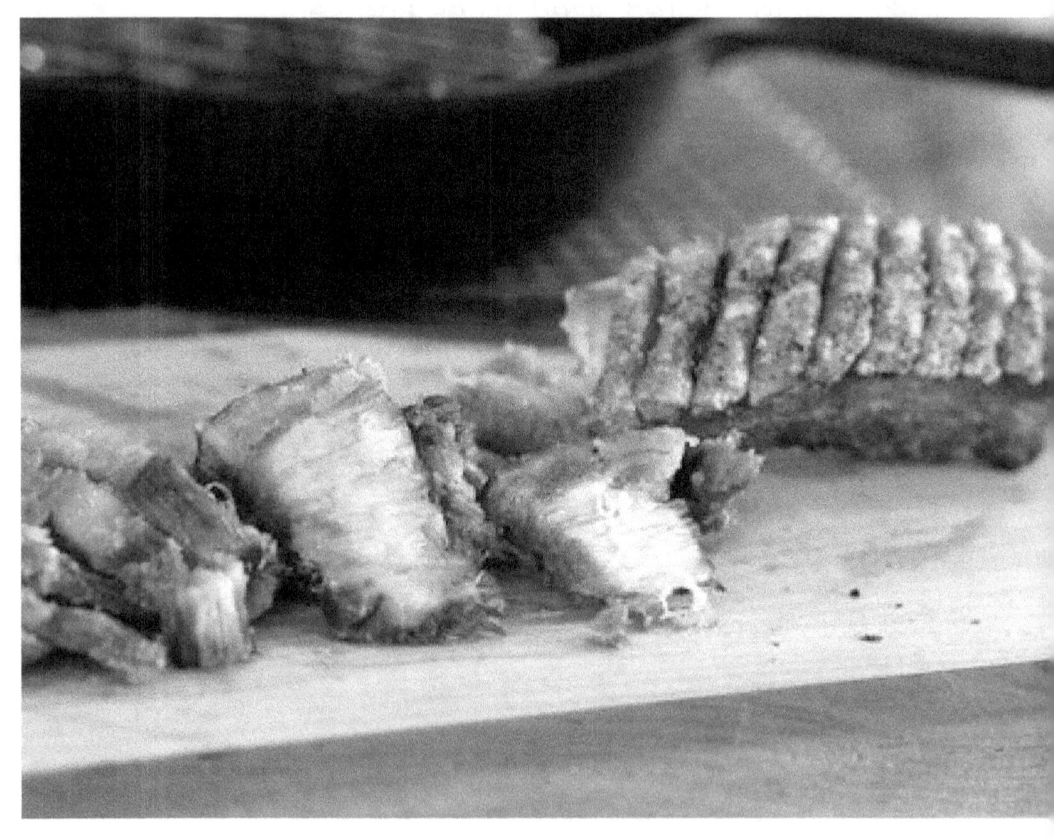

Seasoned Pork Tenderloin

Preparation Time: 10 minutes

Cooking Time: 45 minutes

Servings: 5

Ingredients:

- 1½ pounds pork tenderloin
- 2-3 tablespoons BBQ pork seasoning

Directions:

1. Rub the pork with seasoning generously.

2. Insert the rotisserie rod through the pork tenderloin.

3. Insert the rotisserie forks, one on each side of the rod, to secure the pork tenderloin.

4. Arrange the drip pan at the bottom of the Air Fryer Oven cooking chamber.

5. Select "Roast" and then adjust the temperature to 360 degrees F.

6. Set the timer for 45 minutes and press the "Start."

7. When the display shows "Add Food," press the red lever down and load the rod's left side into the Vortex.

8. Now, slide the rod's left side into the groove along the metal bar, so it doesn't move.

9. Then, close the door and touch "Rotate."

10. When cooking time is complete, press the red lever to release the rod.

11. Remove the pork from Vortex and place it onto a platter for about 10 minutes before slicing.

12. With a sharp knife, cut the roast into desired sized slices and serve.

Nutrition:

Calories 195

Total Fat 4.8 g

Saturated Fat 1.6 g

Cholesterol 99 mg

Sodium 116 mg

Total Carbs 0 g

Fiber 0 g

Sugar 0 g

Protein 35.6 g

Basil Meatloaf With Parmesan

Preparation Time: 40 minutes

Cooking time: 65 minutes

Servings: 5

Ingredients:

- 1cup tomato basil sauce, divided in 2
- 1½ lb. ground beef
- 1¼ cup diced onion
- 2 tbsp. minced garlic
- 2 tbsp. minced ginger
- ½ cup breadcrumbs
- ½ cup grated Parmesan cheese
- Salt and black pepper to taste to season
- 2 tsp. cayenne pepper
- ½ tsp. dried basil

- ⅓   cup chopped parsley

- Two egg whites

Directions:

1. Preheat the Air Fryer to 360 F. In a bowl, add the beef, half of the tomato sauce, onion, garlic, ginger, breadcrumbs, cheese, salt, pepper, cayenne pepper, dried basil, parsley, and egg whites; mix well.

2. Grease an eight or 10-inch pan with cooking spray and scoop the meat mixture into it. Shape the meat into the pan while pressing firmly.

3. Brush the remaining tomato sauce onto meat. Place the pan in the fryer basket and close the Air Fryer; cook for 25 minutes. After 15 minutes, open the fryer, and use a meat thermometer to ensure the meat has reached 160 F internally. If not, cook further for 5 minutes.

4. Remove the pan; drain any excess liquid and fat. Let meatloaf cool for 20 minutes before slicing. Serve with a side of sautéed green beans.

Homemade Beef Liver Soufflé

Preparation Time: 40 minutes

Servings: 4

Ingredients:

- ½ lb. of beef liver

- Three eggs

- 3 oz. buns

- 1cup warm milk

- Salt and black pepper to taste

Directions:

1. Cut the liver into slices and put it in the fridge for 15 minutes. Divide the buns into pieces and soak them in milk for 10 minutes.

2. Put the liver in a blender; add the yolks, the bread mixture, and the spices. Grind

the components and stuff in the ramekins.

3. Line the ramekins in the Air Fryer's basket; cook for 20 minutes at 350 F.

Rib Eye Steak With Avocado Sauce

Preparation Time: 15 minutes

Cooking time: 50 minutes

Servings: 4

Ingredients:

- 1½ lb. rib-eye steak

- 2 tsp. olive oil

- 1 tbsp. chipotle chili pepper

- Salt and black pepper to taste

- One avocado, diced

- Juice from ½ lime

Directions:

1. Place the steak on a chopping board. Pour the olive oil over and sprinkle with the chipotle pepper, salt, and black pepper. Use your hands to rub the spices on the meat. Leave it to sit and marinate for 10

minutes.

2. Preheat the Air Fryer to 400 F. Pull out the fryer basket and place the meat inside. Slide it back into the Air Fryer and cook for 14 minutes. Turn the steak and continue cooking for 6 minutes. Remove the steak, cover with foil, and let it sit for 5 minutes before slicing.

3. Meanwhile, prepare the avocado salsa by mashing the avocado with potato mash. Add in the lime juice and mix until smooth. Taste, adjust the seasoning, slice, and serve with salsa.

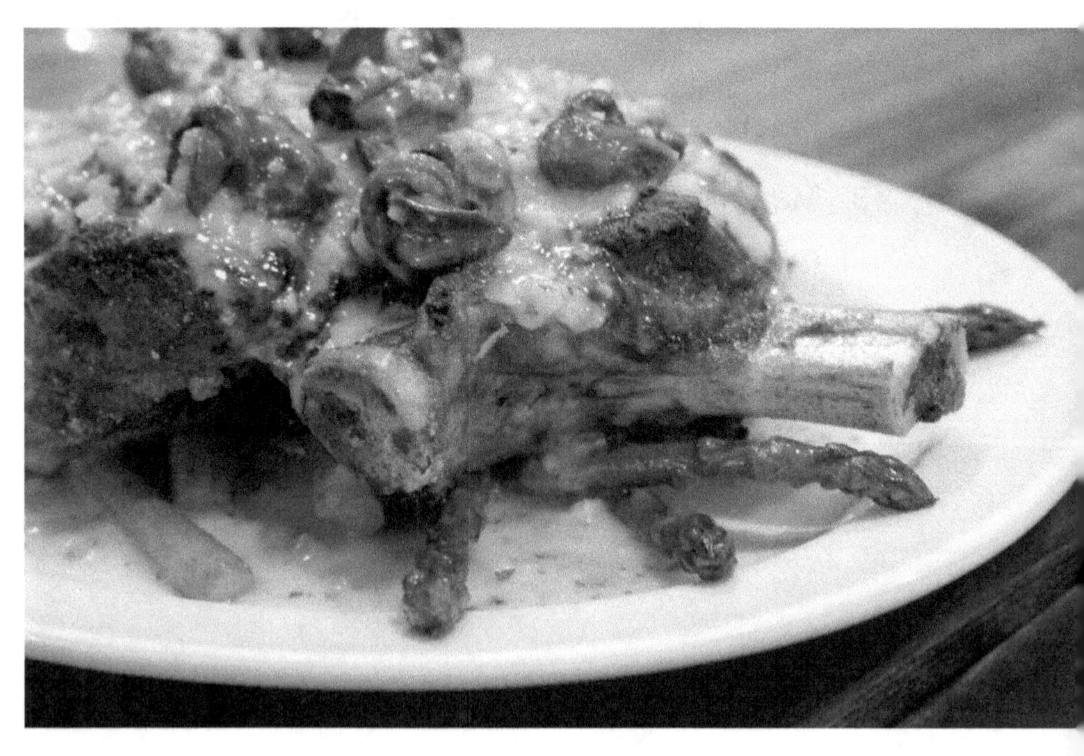